EPILEPSY LESSONS FOR INDEPENDENT LIVING SERIES

Book One: Taking Time to Process Post Diagnosis

Marianne Fehr

A Mouse Nibbles Publication

ISBN 978-1-7773636-0-4

Cover design by: Deven Stanley Wilson

Printed in the United States of America

Acknowledgements

*I would like to acknowledge the people who inspired
and encouraged me to write this series.
Kudos to the people who inspired this book and
encouraged me to write a book on what I have
learnt. Now that will take a bit of doing so I will be
doing a series on the different areas of adjustments
I have had to make. Huge thanks and gratitude go
out to the entire Temporal Lobe Epilepsy (Simple/
Partial Complex Seizures) Facebook group.*

Epigraph

Immediately following my epilepsy diagnosis was an incredible challenge for me. Before I knew I had epilepsy and a few other 'brain challenges', I was freely enjoying life like anyone else in the world. I was going about my regular life when I started noticing that my headaches were growing more frequent– as was the accompanying irritability, drowsiness and lack of energy. I'm telling you, I was getting kinda concerned because it had been going on for at least a year or more. Finally, with some encouragement from a very dear friend, I made the appointment to talk to the doctor about it.

I was suddenly seeing mental health professionals, going for counselling, having bloodwork run– the list goes on. It took over six months of waiting to see the neurologist, then another six months between MRI, EEG & CT scans. It was a nightmare. After the tests were all done, I was stuck waiting again. Having adjusted to being in limbo. I was finally ready for my results, or so I thought.

This is where all the 'fun' begins. Yep, you guessed it, I have epilepsy. But wait, there's more! "Wait! What do you mean there's more?" Well, you could have knocked me over with a butterfly at that point. There I was expecting to hear that the whole thing was a waste of time, like all the other appointments I'd had in the past two years.

What was more is that my neurologist suspected that I was born with brain damage according to the results. He was right about that. I learned from my mama that we had been in an accident in 1962, three months before I was born. Her head went through the windshield while mine went into the dashboard, glove compartment. We had the usual side-effects that go along with a two-vehicle non-rollover type of crash. The doctors told her that she could lose her baby. Well let me tell you, my mama started fighting the doctor on that and told him to never say that to her again. Mama was a true fighter right to the end. Long story short, I was born on February 26th, 1963. Safe to assume I survived just fine.

I was born three months later. Mama recalled to me, "I remember the doctor telling me that I should be grateful that you weren't more brain-damaged than you were." What wasn't taken into account was what kind of brain damage I had or how severe it was. See, when I was born it wasn't just from the car accident that I had brain damage. I got stuck in the birth canal and had to be pushed back in so they could change my position. I had been stuck for over five minutes without oxygen. As you can imagine, that added to my already traumatized brain. This is one of many potential causes of epilepsy. So for me, the hunt was on to discover what else was wrong with me. I still don't know all of it. Some of the mental health issues I have that are directly related to my brain damage. I currently do not have an official diagnosis however, I present with other issues.

That car accident caused damage to my left temporal lobe. We now know this is where my brain damage. Then the doctor goes on to tell me that I have a list of things I am not to be doing anymore. You know the list I'm talking about: the Dos and Don'ts of epilepsy. Well, I needed to find a workaround, being the beautiful multifaceted brained person that I am.

So, you've been diagnosed with epilepsy; welcome to our family. You don't live at home with the folks anymore so you have to learn how to live on your own and be self-sufficient all at the same time. Now that's a blow you were not prepared for, right? I know I was a hot mess when the doctor told me I had epilepsy and would need to turn in my driver's license.

I'd have to say that the biggest pain was hearing that I was no longer allowed to drive. Nor should I have been driving in the first place. I live in the city so I had to learn how to get around using public transportation. So that's no great loss there, right? Not so fast. It's much less expensive to use the public transit system then it is to drive anyway. That being said there is much about one's personal pride at the ability to get where you need to go in your car. It's our independence that takes the hit when we have to stop driving. At least for me.

The need to change was a small "physical" adjustment but the adjustment on the inside of me was like the battle of Armageddon. Our beautiful brains are the real arena. Our brains seem to have this confounded ability to focus on the wrong things.

Well, let's start with the basics of what is going through my head on the day of my original diagnosis and the days following . I was floored, to say the least! I was angry like you wouldn't believe. I vented on the poor doctor who definitely did NOT deserve it. I went outside to cool off & give myself a stern talking to about how you just don't talk to people that way no matter who they are. Then I went back in and apologized to him.

I was never angry with the doctor. I knew he wasn't to blame. I was angrier at the realization that I had been born with a rare form of epilepsy. It has no category because of the complexity of the seizures, the location, the variety of different types of seizures. In fact, about the only thing we know for sure is that it happened 3 months before I was born, due to a car accident my biological parents were in. That's a story for a different series.

CONTENTS

FOREWORD

Epilepsy
Lessons for Independent Living series

I decided to write this series after having conversations with people in a Facebook group that I'm a part of. Many were hinting and suggesting that I write down what I have learned in my epilepsy journey. Thus, the *Lessons for Independent Living* series was born.

I know how hard it can be to make adjustments in your life. Okay, so you can use the word change if you like, but I don't like the word 'change'. I don't know a lot of people who do. For me, the word 'change' has an intense body response. Adjustments is a much more friendly term-it means we just tweak our current course and path of life or what we are doing in our lives. Although we share the same condition we are not all alike. Please keep this in mind if some of the adjustments I have made do not seem to work for you. These are suggestions more than lessons.

My journey since diagnosis has been one filled with learning to live in a way that helps me to live as independently as possible. In all fairness, by the time I found out I had been born with epilepsy caused by brain trauma from a car accident we were in just 3 months prior to my birth. While Mama and I were in the hospital getting checked out the doctor told my Mama she had to be careful or she would lose me. Here a new journey has begun.

DISCLAIMER

I do not know everything about Epilepsy or seizure disorders. This is simply my experience that I am sharing with you. I do not make any medical claims or guarantees that what has worked with me will work with you as we are all different people. I am not a PhD in any form.

SAFETY FIRST

We need to take time to process post-diagnosis in order to give our grey matter time to understand and process this new information. Our brains are filled with neurons, neurotransmitters, veins & vessels, assorted liquids that combine to keep our brain functioning at optimal efficiency. Here's the fallacy though, our brains are not functioning at optimal efficiency. It takes time to translate and distribute information. When a diagnosis takes place your brain creates the thoughts so you can respond at all. Up until your neurologist told you that you had a seizure disorder or epilepsy, your brain was functioning on autopilot. Your brain received an alert from your ears indicating new information that demands an immediate response.

So just as our brains need time to tell the rest of the body what to do, we too need to take time to sit down, breathe, maybe even have that cup of coffee that you were told you had to cut back on. As you are calming your body and natural shock impulses down you can also begin to think more clearly. This is the time to grab your favorite organizational tool and start figuring out how to work things out and what this all means for your life. This process can take time. It has taken me nearly four years to get to where I am today. Be patient with yourself so that your stress hormones don't go out of whack and create a seizure in yourself. That would be bad.

The first thing we need to do is make sure that you are safe in your home. Take out all that information the doctor gave you before you left their office and sit down so you can go over it. They gave you a prescription for some anti-seizure drug (ASD) or anti-epilepsy drug (AED) that you need to take accordingly. Did you have it filled right away on your way home? Did you talk to the pharmacist about the effects, side effects, clashes with other medications, what kind of effect it could have on your vital organs? You have just been diagnosed with an incurable condition, you need to be asking questions. Someone told me decades ago that "There is no such thing as a stupid question. If you are asking it is because you don't know. Questions are how we learn." After that everytime someone told me I was asking a stupid question that was my go-to reply.

The first place you need to familiarize yourself with is the Epilepsy Foundation online. They have a lot of resources that I have accessed over the past few years. Many epilepsy support groups are more than happy to share their knowledge and support with you. Yes, I know it's a challenge to reach out and let others know that something is not right in our brain. It was hard for me that's for sure. This brings us to our next point. Deciding who to tell and how much to tell them.

DECIDING WHO TO TELL & HOW MUCH

Deciding who to tell and how much to tell them can be a tough decision and daunting task. We never really know how people in our circle will respond to such news. Some will be grateful that you have an answer. Some people will distance from you believing you to be contagious in some way, which is laughable.

Voluntary disclosure at a place of employment can be dicey too. You have to choose your words carefully. It is wise to have information handy for your employer to help them understand your needs better. That should help them not to freak out or panic about your condition.I would not recommend blurting it out or just a simple matter of fact "Oh, by the way boss, the doctor diagnosed me with epilepsy. I thought you should know." I mean if you were an employer how would you react or respond to that? The shock factor alone is astronomical and could be a cool way to blow your boss's mind, but I don't recommend it. Now rather than calmly discussing it with your boss you have to first get them calm enough to listen to you, right?

Let's face it, you're already nervous to tell your boss because you don't want to lose your job so you have to have a solid plan before you go in. You're likely wondering why even tell your boss if there's a risk of losing your job, right? Well, it lets them see your honesty level for one. It also shows you what your boss is actually like.

Let's have a look at what happens when the boss doesn't want to listen let alone understand what it even means for you to be diagnosed with a seizure disorder of any kind, let alone epilepsy. Honestly, the first question people seem to ask me is, "So you have the funky chicken dance going on now or what?" In other words, "Do you have convulsive seizures?". Not typically, I don't. I do have them if my body is rejecting a particular drug, however that is very rare. I am incredibly cautious about my medications because of an ongoing experience I had as a child.

The point of all this is that some bosses don't even care about what a seizure or epilepsy is, let alone how it affects you so as long as you can do your job. On the other hand, when your boss does understand and wants to learn more about this, it's a fantastic opportunity to educate them and everyone else you work with. You are likely in the early stages of post-diagnosis. If this is the case you will likely have information from the doctors. Maybe even form your boss will need to fill out if you can continue to be gainfully employed. Some employers have amendments in their contracts that allow for situations like ours. These types of bosses are fantastic and usually like to find a way to help you as you are adjusting to a new kind of life. You were open and honest with them about what is really happening and why you haven't been your usual self. The good ones will notice the change in you when you are unwell in any way. These are the bosses to stay with as long as you can.

You might be thinking to yourself, "You said this was going to be a challenge, but I don't see one. Why is this such a delicate dance then?" Well, I'm glad you asked. Not every boss is easy going. You don't want to spit out everything about your health. You are allowed to tell them you don't have an answer yet. Some things need to be shared. Nor is it their business if you have decided to opt for surgery or not until you need to tell them. I think it's a good idea to wait with that until you have the paperwork for your surgery.

So far all I have been talking to you about is your employer. You need to find a way to break this news to your family and friends as well. When you are telling them about your diagnosis please do remember to check, recheck and check again. Not everyone in your circle will handle this information the same. We are all different as evidenced by their response.

Just like with employers, family and friends can get to be a challenge to navigate for a vast variety of reasons. This checking and rechecking is to help you know when enough is enough. Don't let anyone push you if you feel they are asking you to divulge too much.

WORKING OUT TRANSPORTA-TION NEEDS

We are told that we are not permitted to drive until we have been seizure free for a certain amount of time. For you it could be as little as six months. For me, it's six years. Why? Well, my guess is that it could be the rarity of my particular type or placement of the seizure area in my brain. That's my guess. Six months appears to be the standard across the international medical field from what I understand.

This area of our condition appears to be a hotspot for those of us with epilepsy. The first thing we lose is our independence– before we even leave the doctor's office post-diagnosis. It hit me pretty hard when I heard it was likely I wasn't going to be driving again in my lifetime. I needed to get organized fast because I needed to be able to get around in a vehicle to go to places without transit stops. As you can imagine I no longer work in that high-stress job. I was a resident manager of one of the more dangerous apartment buildings in the city.

Once I left that employer I needed to get into a new apartment and get my finances in order. A friend has a place in the bush so I went out there to think without worrying about finances. It was about three months later I had been approved for an apartment within my price range. I still insisted on doing something, anything for work. I was blessed with a very good paying job and since it was a term position I thought I could manage it.

I know not everyone can do what I did to take time to process post-diagnosis. I did not understand for over a year that I was now considered disabled. See, my epilepsy is drug-resistant, uncategorized left temporal lobe simple/complex partial epilepsy. Wow that's a mouthful. Point is, it is due to the rarity and the resistance to drugs pretty much meant I wasn't going to be able to drive again. I had to face facts, it was time to learn the public transit system if I wanted any form of independence.

I can hear you already, I will never take public transportation especially in light of the current pandemic. Well, what can I tell you? Put on your mask, possibly even gloves and roll up your sleeves and put on your boots, it's time to dig in to do what you don't want to do.

Now if you have the cash for it you could use taxis however that will get expensive very quickly. So does having a driving service on call or handy. Again if you have the money to do that I will not hold it against you. If you need more resources on this please check out the resources on Epilepsy Foundation website. I will go into more depth on this in my book Epilepsy Lessons for Independent Living Series, Book Nine: Getting Around; The Mobility Factor. Book Nine will have options and resources for you to access. I have attempted to include universal resources in an effort to help you wherever you live.

OUR HOME, FAMILY, OUR OWN LIVES

Your neurologist and your regular doctor have both likely given you all sorts of information to look through and find a new way of living to adjust to. There are all those things you are suddenly no longer permitted to do. This is what this series is all about; helping people who are diagnosed with a seizure disorder. Even if you have a feeling or suspect it to be an issue for you it never hurts to have this kind of information handy should you need it.

By now you have told your family/roommates or anyone who may be living with or close to you. If you're not ready for this step that is perfectly fine. You are still processing. You are allowed to take as much time as you need. Never rush a decision about your health or your life. Anyone who is trying to push you along is not doing it for your sake. They are doing it for their own sake. It could be they are uncomfortable with the changes and want life to get back to normal. The issue here is, that once you have been diagnosed with any type of seizure disorder, your life has changed and now you have to adjust and adapt to a new way of living and caring for yourself.

The very first thing I had to do was get rid of my coffee table. I kept getting bruises on my legs and didn't know how they were happening. When I told the neurologist he recommended removing any objects from the center of the rooms and to see if that took care of it. Sure enough, the problem was solved.

Now I live with 95% of my hard furniture against the walls and have room to walk so I don't bang into everything. My balance has been off most of my life so I always had bruises everywhere.

We need to look at our home, our friends, our family, our income streams, and our life partners if we have one. Do we have the space to facilitate a yoga mat or a nice area rug that we can do stretches and some workouts on? Do we have things we need to part with to make our home safe for us to be in? "Marianne, why do you make it sound like we're moving?" You're not preparing to move. You are preparing to make your home a safe place for you to be. A stress-free home. I can tell you first hand that for me a mess of any kind, even dishes on the counter can cause me serious stress. Then whoops there is that dang seizure. We have to think about safety first. It doesn't matter what type of seizures you have, what matters is that your home is safe in case you fall while having a seizure. This is all about protecting your brain now. We need our brain so we can live. Our brain tells us to breathe, to eat, to sleep, that we love, that we cry, that we are happy, that we really want something or don't want something. Without our brain our heart would not beat and our blood would stop flowing. We need to protect our brain because it is the most vital organ in our entire body. If it wasn't it would have a shell around the grey matter like it does.

Now stop and breathe for a second. No laughing seizures on my watch, please. We need to be careful with our brain. In this Epilepsy Lessons for Independent Living series I will do my best to cover everything that is important for a safe home. Having a safe home is something most people don't even think about. In a loose sense that is what you will be doing too, baby-proofing the home– but only to a point. No, you don't have to put protective outlet covers into your electrical sockets. Let's not get carried away here; we are adults, after all.

We simply need to ensure that if we have a seizure in bed and we roll onto the floor that we are not hitting the corner of the night table on the way out of bed. You can have a night table, that's not what I am saying at all. I'm saying think about the placement of your hard furniture. I will definitely be going into further detail on this in Epilepsy Lessons for Independent Living series Book Three: Self Care and

Housework.

YOUR HAMSTER
IS WORKING
TOO FAST

Yes, that is what I said. Your hamster is working too fast. You just got bombarded with shocking, life-changing information.

We all need time to process after receiving a diagnosis. Some things don't require as much downtime as other issues. For example: suppose you have found out that you were just having headaches because you weren't drinking enough water. Well, that doesn't take time to process. Just make a conscious effort to drink more water. However, since you have just recently been diagnosed with epilepsy. It's gonna take some time, some planning and even some relaxation techniques to get through your first little while. Getting things sorted out and working correctly for you and your life will take time. At this point, it doesn't matter what anyone else wants you to do. This is your life, your brain that we are talking about here and that is solely your decision. This is you taking care of you. I will go more in depth on this in my book Epilepsy Lessons for Independent Living Series, Book Three: Self Care And Housework.

The risks of making snap treatment choices immediately following diagnosis can mess up our lives. Especially if we take a treatment option because someone else wants us to, not because we chose to.

We need time to cool down after a shock. Emergency Medical Services won't let you leave after something shocking until you are okay or have someone with you who is responsible enough to care for your needs until the end of the shock period.

As you can see clarity of mind is a necessity from the start. We need to take this time to allow our brain to process this shocking information it has received.

See, one of the hardest things for me to do was find time to calm down enough to process. I left that neurologist's office without him realizing that I was in a full-on rage seizure, but I digress. Now if I had taken someone with me, anyone, then I would have been able to process easier. Unfortunately for me at that time, I didn't know the young lady that I know now. She would have gone with me to every appointment, made sure I knew all my options and if the dosages were too high from the onset. That's another thing, do not let them give you the highest dosage first. Start low and work up.

DECIDING ON
THE BEST GAME
PLAN FOR **YOU**

T he hardest thing you may have to deal with is the realization that you may have to adjust your current life plan. This is a new phase of living independently and you will need to have a solid plan in place. This could be time-consuming and even somewhat challenging but have no fear. I know you can do this. If I can you can too.

When you talk to your core circle of friends and family, have your information handy so you can answer your circle as they are likely to ask lots of questions. You want to be able to answer them to the best of your ability. This will also help you learn what all you actually will need to adjust, alter and/ or forgo from here on in. It is also wise to check out all the resources available to you on the Epilepsy Foundation website. I have noticed that they allow global access as well as country-specific searching and information on the site. Your regular doctor should be able to direct you as well. Take any and all information that is provided for you. This too will help you educate yourself and those around you.

I'm one of those private people who did 95% of this alone. I looked everything up on my own. I chose when to tell family members and friends. Some people I just blurted it out and left them in shock. Some people left my life because they were scared or unwilling to make the needed effort to try to understand. My family however was a totally different story. My youngest sister was like, "Now that explains a lot." My mama & daddy were both calm, cool and collected. Mama was a little quieter. I'm not sure what she was thinking but I have to wonder if she blamed herself for not finding out when I was little. She said she knew something was off because the teachers kept sending her notes or calling her at work. Saying things such as, "Marianne is not following instructions in class." "Marianne is not paying attention in class." "Marianne is daydreaming in class." ...You get the idea.

NEUROLOGIST FOLLOW-UP APPOINTMENTS WHY FOLLOW-UP IS KEY

The first appointment after a test that reveals seizure activity is very important. "It's important to make a follow-up appointment with your neurologist. This appointment is for asking questions about your condition/s and options. If you're comfortable having someone come with you to listen, I'd recommend it." Most of the time there is no problem with this. Now, I'm a little too independent for my own good. For me it's a challenge asking anyone to help with pretty much anything. Now that you have booked a follow-up appointment, you have time to discuss your options with your core circle of people and you have to ask just one person to attend with you. This was a huge error on my part. I should have asked someone, anyone, to attend with me.

At this appointment, all you are doing is discussing your options and what they entail. The doctors seem to always reach for the prescription pad but that's not always the best route to take, as is my case. There are a few types of surgeries that I know about that have proven successful for some people. I have chosen for myself that many may not comprehend and that's okay by me. I will not be having surgeries at all for my epilepsy. I can't take the meds so that leaves one thing, my diet and lifestyle choices.

Wait, but Marianne you just said surgeries can be successful. Yes, I did. I also said this was my choice. See I am donating my brain to the Epilepsy and Seizure Foundation so that they can research my particular type of rare epilepsy. As I said earlier, mine is uncategorized. That means they don't know what type of issues caused the damage to my brain or where it puts me in the grand scheme of things. For me, that is a perfect opportunity to help other people like me. I love helping people whenever and wherever I can. For the best way for them to figure out how to stop these kinds of things happening to someone else is to be able to have a frame of reference. That's what I'm doing, giving them a "virgin brain" to work with.

Make and attend one more follow-up appointment

and present your decision to the neurologist so that they can get the ball rolling on whatever your treatment needs are. These appointments should be as close together as possible. Usually a week or two from the date you attended your diagnosis appointment.

NO CURE FOR EPILEPSY **YET**

The harsh reality that we are living with an incurable condition, for now. I think that we, as a global community, need to start brainstorming together. How can we discover a cure for our seizures so that we can help the next generation of people with epilepsy or a seizure disorder?

Yes, we can try to modify the Ketogenic Diet plan or just eat fruit and vegetables. For many that can work. If it was just a matter of food the only people who would be diagnosed would be the ones who could afford to get tested and treated. That's not fair. It sets up a line of discrimination and prejudice. I think we can all agree that we have no place in our community for that. We don't need more division in our global community.

As a global community, we could put all our heads together and come up with solutions that would benefit us who currently struggle already and the generations to come. Ideally, we would be better served to come up with a plan or method for not having our beautifully created brains damaged in the first place.

Let me take a short bunny trail here.

I love my brain. I say "our beautifully created brains" because we need to also see that our damaged brain has given us both a curse (the seizures) and a blessing. We have access to both sides of our brains! Think about that for a second. Okay, take another second to think about that. Most people only have access to one hemisphere, but we have both hemispheres at our disposal. So if we, who have access to our entire brain not only half of it, then I think we can find something that could help everyone across the board. What do you think?

SUDDEN UNEXPECTED DEATH IN EPILEPSY

The risk of Sudden Unexpected Death in Epilepsy (SUDEP) is very small, but there is a risk nonetheless. We as persons with epilepsy and seizure disorders could have alarm bells going off inside of us like emergency lights. Stop. There is no need to panic about this realization. Everyone runs the risk of not waking up from their slumber. Do not let this become a paralyzing fear for you. All fear does is create a higher chance for a seizure to occur so we must stay as calm as possible. Not giving into the fatalistic mentality is important. There may be no cure but it doesn't have to crush us. We do not need to allow this to cause us to feel like there is no point in going on.

I find it necessary to include this small, yet intimidating piece of information. It is noteworthy for adding into your affairs in order. Yep, that's right. I'm talking about death prep while talking about SUDEP. Why on earth would I bring that up after telling you that we can die in our sleep after a seizure? Well, to be honest with you, it's a reality – albeit an unpleasant one that no one wants to discuss. Death is a part of living.

Why do I mention bringing it up in your affairs in order? Do you want your funeral held up because the police have decided that you died under suspicious circumstances? I didn't think so. Well, then it has to be included in your living will, that it is a very real possibility and to check for it first during an autopsy. Yeah okay, this is kinda morbid. I'll give you that. But do you want to have this kind of conversation with your kids, your life partner or the nurses at the hospital while you lay on your deathbed at the tender age of 125 years young? Well, if you're like me you want to keep some things private. I know I have become much more private since I was diagnosed. Oh, I told my family and likely drove them nuts with it all.

From what I understand, the numbers are incredibly low for SUDEP to happen. Out of the entire global epilepsy community, The number is in the range of 0.1 – 0.3% of all of us who have been diagnosed with epilepsy. Let's put that into a fraction just for the sake of understanding. 1/1,000. This is completely hypothetical numbers so please, to be accurate check the Epilepsy Foundation online. I will include the link in the reference area of this book.

As you can see it is a very tiny percentage of people who will die of SUDEP. Now that we have that established please take a few calming deep breaths and relax. A glass of water will help your neurons to calm as well. Yep, I said water. Water is one of the healthiest things you can put into your body, once it's been filtered that is. Drinking pond water without boiling and triple filtration is not healthy.

Now that you are relaxed again let us recap just a touch. SUDEP is extremely rare but because it might happen, I deemed it worth mentioning. The one thing I would recommend is that you talk to both your neurologist, your regular doctor. Your pharmacist about any other health issues you have to know just how much of a risk you are at. We all have different health issues that need to be taken into account with epilepsy and seizure disorders. There may be overlapping symptoms, drug reactions that could be triggering the seizures. Your pharmacist can answer your questions about drug interactions, complications and where overdosing can occur. So make sure you talk to them about your questions.

THE NEXT STEP FOR INDEPENDENT LIVING

This is where the rest of the series comes in. I have decided to break it down into bite-sized pieces to make it easier on you. I go into a lot of detail on how to do things that you enjoy doing and how to do them safely.

Living alone vs living with others will largely be age-dependent and dependent upon your strengths, weaknesses and resources available to you. Some people will let their homecare workers know about the changes and they will do the rest after that. Some people are barely moved out from home and either working or in continuing education. All these factors and many more need to be taken into account before you make that decision.

Your time immediately post-diagnosis is important and filled to overflowing with choices, decisions, alterations and adjustments that you have to cope with. Understand that when I say this I am not saying that you have to change 100% of the way you live– far from it. It's more about awareness, being present in your surroundings and living your life in the safest way possible while still enjoying living your life as independently as possible.

Many people make the mistake of assuming that a diagnosis is the end of the world. Well, that is only partly true. It is the end of the old world you are accustomed to, but it is also a beginning. "Marianne are you completely crazy? What do you mean it's a beginning? I just got the devastating news that I have an incurable condition and you are saying it's a beginning?" No, I am not crazy.

I want you to consider this; yes you just got your diagnosis. No, you are not feeling okay because your brain is busy trying to find a way to calm you down so that it can help you think and process. This does not happen overnight. It takes time so permit yourself to take this time just for you. If you have to go sit in the bathroom with the door locked. Perhaps have the shower on while you read, pray or whatever it is you need to do for you can think clearer. It has taken me four years to adapt and adjust my life to fit my particular safety levels.

"In the unlikely event of an emergency,
Don't Panic.
Defrost the fridge."

SM Fehr
(My Mama)

"How do I adjust to living independently in my family?" Now that is a good question is it not? Well for starters, this depends on your age and which family you refer to. If you are the kind of person who thinks they can handle living alone, try it. However, if you are attached I would recommend a family meeting without digital devices in hands if at all possible. If you need to, turn it into a special family meal. Go ahead and plan it so it fits in with your family's busy schedule.

If you cannot get your entire family together in one place you can get them all together in a conference call style of your choosing. Now it is wise to have your information handy so that you can answer as many of their questions as possible. If you do not know the answer to a question do not hesitate to say so and remind them that you are also learning with them.

"How do I tell my family about adjustments?" That is a good question, and one that only you have the answer to. I recommend taking your time, sitting down with your loved ones, and being honest. It is wise to have some information handy so that you can answer as many of their questions as possible.

Your family needs to be able to access the same educational aids you are using. This will help educate them on what to do when, how and why. We need to educate our family and friends when they are willing to learn.

You should be prepared to lose friends. Not everyone will understand or want to be around you if you cannot join in with their idea of fun. I have lost some friends but I have made many many more much closer and dearer friends in support groups. I would like to recommend that you find a support group online that will help you through the adjustment process. New patients are always joining us and asking about different medication effects that people have had, side effects they experienced and if it is even the correct type of medication or treatment for them. We share funny things, struggles, question and answer sessions are sometimes held. We all share what we have learned with everyone else in the group. In this way, we grow together and as individuals.

Epilepsy Lessons for Independent Living Series, Book One: Taking Time to Process Post Diagnosis is only the first book in this series. In the rest of the series, we will be looking at everything from soup to nuts and much more in much greater detail. Well, at least as far as my personal experience goes. I will also be including resources for you to access and use. "How do I tell my family about adjustments?" That is a good question, and one that only you have the answer to. I recommend taking your time, sitting down with your loved ones, and being honest. It is wise to have some information handy so that you can answer as many of their questions as possible.

EPILOGUE

Epilepsy Lessons for Independent Living Series, Book One: Taking Time to Process Post Diagnosis is only the first book in this series. In the rest of the series, we will be looking at everything from soup to nuts and much more in much greater detail. Well, at least as far as my personal experience goes. I will also be including resources for you to access and use. "How do I tell my family about adjustments?" That is a good question, and one that only you have the answer to. I recommend taking your time, sitting down with your loved ones, and being honest. It is wise to have some information handy so that you can answer as many of their questions as possible.

AFTERWORD

I'd say let's start at the top and work our way down.... but I have a different plan of attack in this series. In this series I'm going to start with a few of our hot spots or triggers if you will. So, shall we dig in and get on with it or would you like to grab your favorite book reading items first? Epilepsy: Lessons for Independent Living Series: Book One: Taking Time to Process Post Diagnosis is intended to be a bit of an opener to the rest of the series. In future books we will be looking at everything from cooking to relationships and everything in between.

ACKNOWLEDGEMENT

*I would like to take a moment
to express my gratitude to
Deven Stanley Wilson for
designing the book cover
and editing of this book.*

*I would also like to thank my 'Pre-launch Review
Team' for doing reviews on Epilepsy: Lessons
for Independent Living Series: Book One:
Taking Time to Process Post Diagnosis.*

ABOUT THE AUTHOR

Marianne Fehr

Mariannne Fehr has lived for more than 50 years without being aware of epilepsy. Ms Fehr has not considered Epilepsy as a hindrance to living a fully independent life. Marianne was raised in the country area of the prairies of southern Manitoba. This instilled in her a strong sense of independence. Marianne has never backed down from a challenge. Marianne has occasionally, yet seriously stated, "I'll figure this out yet. I just need time. I'll figure it out yet, you'll see." Due to her tenacity, Marianne achieves whatever she sets her mind to. Having this in mind and with specific encouragement Ms Fehr decided to write the Epilepsy Lessons for Independent Living series. Ms Fehr speaks from the heart and encourages others to remember that they are not alone and they can do something that they have been told they can't.

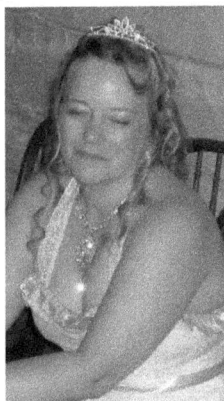

https://mousenibbles2020.blogspot.com
https://www.facebook.com/mjoy.fehr

EPILEPSY LESSONS FOR INDEPENDENT LIVING SERIES

Epilepsy can be rough if you don't know what to expect. This is one woman's personal journey from blissfully unaware to finding a way to live independently of others. Personal independence can make the difference between giving up and moving forward in life.

Epilepsy Lessons For Independent Living Series Book One: Taking Time To Process

The need to take time to process hinders the fear monster in the closet.

Epilepsy Lessons For Independent Living Series Book Two: Cooking; Finding A Practical Work Around

Debunking the "No Cooking" mentality. There's

more than one way to bring a tree down. Cooking with Epilespy is just another tree that needs to be removed from the view.

Epilepsy Lessons For Independent Living Series Book Three: Self Care And Housework

Self care has been a very prominent thing in our society in the past decade or so. Citing mental health as a key factor for self care.
As with housework, self care can easily be added to any daily routine according to one's personal abilities.

Bedroom Stuffepilepsy Lessons For Independent Living Series Book Four: That No One Wants To Talk About. Hormones, Sex And Seizures

The big 'taboo' conversations that no one really wants to talk about.

Epilepsy Lessons For Independent Living Series Book Five: Movies, Concerts, Strobe Lights And Games; What's The Deal?

Logical reasons for doctors saying that movies, concerts, strobe lights and the like should be avoided. We will get into the deal on that.

Epilepsy Lessons For Independent Living Series Book Six: Anxiety And Social Situations

Anxiety and social situations take many things into account that can and does cause some people triggers for different types of seizures.

Epilepsy Lessons For Independent Living Series Book Seven: Pets, Service Animals And Why They Are Important

Important roles of the feline and canine community and how they can help us feel safe.

Epilepsy Lessons For Independent Living Series Book Eight: Relationships: Ugh! Can We Please Talk About Anything Else? Why I Chose To Be Single

The difficult discussion on relationships and why this author decided to stay single.

Epilepsy Lessons For Independent Living Series Book Nine: Getting Around: The Mobility Factor And Safety Pro's

And Con's

Mobility and personal independence seem to be linked.

Epilepsy Lessons For Independent Living Series Book Ten: Pain, Medications And Other Complications

Pain, Medications And Other Complications explores the reasons behind things that work for some but not all.

Epilepsy Lessons For Independent Living Series Book Eleven: Dreams, Ambitions And Reclaiming Your Life

Inspiration to help you start fighting back for your life, well being and revealing that you still have dreams, ambitions, goals and desires.

Epilepsy Lessons For Independent Living Series Book Twelve: Are You Ready To Live Your Best Life? Yes You Can!

Helping you as I have been helped.

www.ingramcontent.com/pod-product-compliance
Lightning Source LLC
Chambersburg PA
CBHW060642280326
41933CB00012B/2122